MW01016348

the devi of speech

the goddess in kundalini yoga

the devi of speech

swami sivananda radha

with a foreword
by swami radhananda

timeless books
www.timeless.org
©2005 timeless books

cover design by todd stewart
interior design by colin dorsey
cover photo by andrea rollefson
This edition is printed in Canada on 80% recycled, 20% post
consumer waste paper that is chlorine and acid free.

Library and Archives Canada Cataloguing in Publication

Radha, Swami Sivananda, 1911-1995. The Devi of Speech :
The Goddess in Kundalini Yoga/Swami Sivananda Radha.
Includes bibliographical references.   ISBN 1-932018-06-9
1. Kundalini.   2. Devi.   3. Meditation.   1. Title.
BL1238.56.K86R32   2005   294.5'436   C2005-900827-S

Also by Swami Sivananda Radha

Books

Mantras: Words of Power (2005)
When You First Called Me Radha: Poems (2005)
Kundalini Yoga for the West (2004)
Realities of the Dreaming Mind (2004)
Radha: Diary of a Woman's Search (2002)
Time to be Holy (1996)
Hatha Yoga: The Hidden Language (1995)
From the Mating Dance to the Cosmic Dance (1992)
In the Company of the Wise (1991)

Timeless Small Book Series

The Rose Ceremony (2004)
The Divine Light Invocation: A Healing Meditation (2001)

contents

Foreword

In the practice of Kundalini Yoga, speech is sometimes represented as a goddess who is known as Sakti or the Devi of Speech. The Devi of Speech has the power to bring understanding and insights. She is the bridge that connects us to what is happening within and what is manifesting outwardly. This book is about the Goddess, Her Power and its importance in our spiritual development.

Much of the material is excerpted from Swami Radha's *Kundalini Yoga for the West*, an intensive work that translates the ancient mysteries of Kundalini into practical tools for self-study and character building. The focus of this book is exclusively on the Devi. Swami Radha would often instruct her students to follow the thread of the Goddess, saying, "The Devi of Speech is one of the most important parts of the *Kundalini* book." By concentrating on her writings about the Devi, we can begin to understand how the feminine creative force is constantly at work in our lives.

The study of Kundalini is the study of the Devi — the study of your Self. The Goddess gives the teachings that will take you from the limited ideas of life to expanded, limitless vistas.

The Kundalini system, very simply, is a map of the seven levels of consciousness, with each level or *cakra* pictured as a lotus. Every lotus petal of each cakra is inscribed with one of the 52 letters of the Sanskrit alphabet. The letters are called *matrikas* or "little mothers" because the letters give birth to language and language creates our perception of the world. The letters are imbued with power, and this unmanifest energy has to manifest in order to be known, just as ideas and thoughts are made visible in our speech and actions.

A form of the Devi or Sakti is also present in each cakra. She represents the intelligence and creativity at every level of awareness and the ever evolving power of speech. Within each person is the seed of Divine potential – Kundalini – and we can use speech to develop awareness of that potential. The more we know about ourselves and the greater our awareness, the more we can make conscious choices of who we want to be and what we want to create in the world.

Swami Radha's own investigation of the Devi was particularly inspired by the *Ananda Lahari* or *The Wave of Bliss*, ancient verses in praise of Divine Mother.[1] A few of those verses play a large role in this book, in particular, the mantras describing each cakra.

Swami Radha studied these verses to deepen her own understanding of the Divine Feminine. She encourages us to use these mantras to find our own way to the Devi: "The cream of all the Teachings, in regards to the Devi of Speech, are the Kundalini mantras. You need to absorb yourself in these mantras. My commentary can only be a guideline for how you can get your own insights. What are they saying? Within them are many answers. Write your own commentary."

Through your own investigation you can discover and uncover the unique meanings of the Kundalini system. In *The Devi of Speech*, we explore the Goddess cakra by cakra, using reflection exercises and meditations on Divine Mother. There is a focus on the Divine Mother prayer, a simple and powerful mantra, also taken from the *Ananda Lahari*. By practising this mantra you affirm that everything you do is worship of Divine Mother, that every natural function and action is a form of worship. It is a continuous offering. Through dedication, humility, surrender and the sincere desire to know ourselves, we can bring the words to life. This is the promise of the Goddess.

O ver years of using these reflections and exercises with students, I have seen the care with which the Devi manifests, as people face the obstacles in their lives with teachings that allow them to see their own inner strength. I have heard the Devi in moments of inspiration and joy, in moments of pain, and in the deepest doubt and grieving as we learn about our human condition. If you listen carefully and are attentive, speech provides very immediate feedback on what is happening both personally and in the situations around you. The words people use are so present and personal to what is happening, and together we can learn to listen to the elements of speech, audible and inaudible.

This kind of awareness will begin to move you beyond the ignorance that keeps you bound. And that is the compassion of Divine Mother. She always gives us another chance, no matter what our situation in life is, if we pursue our desire for self-awareness with sincerity. Devotion to the Goddess, coming from the heart, will bring liberation.

The mystery is to see Her in action, to recognize Her in the world, and in yourself. "She is the energy in the sun, the fragrance in the flowers, the beauty in the landscape. She is the primal life force that underlies all existence."[2]

Her mystery is very precious. The work you put into learning more about your own mystery is precious. In the *Devi Gita*,[3] the Goddess cautions,

"Do not reveal this secret mystery that I have narrated to just anybody, anywhere. Diligently guard the secret mystery of this song."

It will take effort to reveal your own mystery, but persistence leads to self-realization.

— Swami Radhananda
Yasodhara Ashram, May 2005

1   Swami Siyananda (trans.), *Ananda Lahari* (*The Wave of Bliss*), Calcutta, India: The S.P. League, 1949.

2   Swami Sivananda Radha, *Kundalini Yoga for the West*, Kootenay Bay, BC: Timeless Books, 2004.

3   C. Mackenzie Brown, *Devi Gita: Song of the Goddess*, Albany, NY: SUNY Press, 1998.

the devi

O Devi! O Sarasvati!
Reside Thou ever in my speech.
Reside Thou ever on my tongue tip.
O Divine Mother, giver of faultless poetry.

sakti power: energy manifest

Sakti is the Great Mother. In glory She surpasses a father at all times. Mother Sakti holds the child, the seeker, the aspirant in Her womb, which is the world. She nourishes the child with Divine nectar, which brings the child back to Mother, after the enjoyment of the play of Maya.

All practice in Kundalini Yoga must be understood as an approach to the Devi. Sakti is the origin of all. Sakti is the source. Whatever one worships and admires, it is Sakti. She is the form, the ideal, the Power — the Goddess of the spoken word. It is for this reason that Sakti is also life, breath — existence itself. Sakti is one Power becoming many. All that is manifest has an innate power that is from the same source. There is one sun having many rays. All rays emanate from the source.

Sakti's Power is the manifestation of the microcosmos as well as the macrocosmos. Sakti is all the Power there is to be experienced. She is called the Devi of Speech, the whisper that is in every illusion. She is also the thunder of the Cosmic voice.

The two extreme gifts that one can obtain from Divine Mother are Her Maya (continuous illusion) and Liberation from the bondage of all illusion. Each human experience is at some point on the sweep between these extremes of Maya and Liberation. The movement of every human life shows the intermingling of countless possibilities. Only by a decisive act of will can we stop running all over the place. Remember, by the manifestation of Her Power is this whole universe set in motion — revolving, moving constantly.

Femininity and masculinity exist wherever there is creation. The ancient texts call the male Divine Force the Deva and the female the Devi, in accordance with the male and female principle in all fathers and mothers in the world. Energy per se is symbolized in the male aspect. Energy manifest is symbolized in the female aspect.

How can Energy be known? Its presence is recognized in its manifestations. The old yogis stated that Energy and its manifestations are inseparable. Some texts refer to that Energy as Light, some use the Mother as symbol – She gives birth to the child. Energy gives birth to various creations. She is the Great Mother. As the Mother of all, She is Sakti. This is a simple way to explain what cannot be said in the words that are used in daily communication. This is poetic expression, and poetry is the language of inspiration.

In order to understand Sakti Power it is necessary that one recognize power in its most simple manifestations. Electricity is a familiar energy. It is easy for the mind to understand its physical forms, such as a light, a heater or a running motor. The light and the heater can be seen as concrete symbols of electricity. But the mind needs a particular training to understand beyond the symbols. The difficulties become apparent when we practise thinking of ourselves without the body or face – we are familiar with ourselves and often even quite emphatic about what we know of ourselves, but can we conceptualize ourselves beyond the physical?

We can use these illustrations and carry them a step further. To understand terms like "God," the "Absolute" and "Cosmic Energy," special training and new experiences are necessary. How can we otherwise overcome the old familiar process of creating and recreating the Absolute or God in our own image and even adding human characteristics to it, however perfect these may be?

In Eastern thought, God is understood as Energy manifesting in many aspects. The mind and its many possible manifestations are an expression of that one Power.

One of the greatest powers we have, although it is often not recognized, is the power of choice. With our mental power, we can choose to be kind, understanding and helpful, or jealous, envious and destructive. We can choose to give or to steal. The polarity is within us, and we first have to recognize it and then take responsibility for both the positive and negative ways we handle our power.

We evolve spiritually through our own personal efforts to understand the power that keeps us alive, the power that makes our minds work. As we grow in awareness, we start to understand more of that Cosmic Power. In India the name given to that Power is Kundalini. In Greece it is called the "soul." Nobody has seen either. We can't always see everything, but just as in physics, we can see the traces. By starting to get to know ourselves and tracing the events of our lives, we will begin to see ourselves on a different scale than we are used to.

So ask yourself: What power am I engaging? What power am I loosening? If you have no control over it, what good is it? You have to go through life with awareness, thinking things through. Self-discipline and foresight are needed. If you want the Power of Kundalini, of the Devi, you have to think it through. How do you use the powers you already have? Only you are responsible for your actions.

exploring the devi

When we investigate something, we have to start at the bottom and move our way up so that we really understand what it means. The *Devi of Speech*. What do we mean by this? *Devi* stands really for the word *Power*, the power of speech. And before we think about the power of speech, we have to look at the human voice.

The human voice is an instrument, whose impact we should not overlook. There is no musical instrument created that has the same power as the human voice. The way you talk, the way you use your voice and your breath, by saying just one word you can express as many emotions as there are keys on the keyboard of a grand piano. In fact, there is no emotion that you can't express through your voice; even if you suppress your voice, it comes through your breath.

In the yogic tradition there is a distinction made between emotions and feelings. Feelings are cultivated emotions. When we cultivate our emotions, they become refined feelings, and we are capable of having a certain warmth in our voice, a certain softness and loving tone. We can kindle hope in another person in the way we say something, express our consideration, our concern. The voice can become very melodious and clear. You can also see the opposite, that when the voice is vibrating with emotions it is everything but steady.

The way in which we use our voice, we can realize we have tremendous power. We can shake somebody up. And we can also elevate somebody. We can see that the human voice has a range from very low to very high, and vice versa. When we speak, our own voice can tell us where we are at, at any given moment.

The human voice is then a bridge between two worlds — not only between your lower nature and your highest nature, but also between a world of chatter and one of utter silence. Such an absolute silence we can acquire in the practice of meditation.

When we are in this silence, we can become quite

aware of the vibrations of our sound, the sound of our voice. We know when we sigh, we know when we take a deep breath, and we may hear the sound of the heart. We may have an urge to speak, but this great silence embraces us, and we find it superfluous to even say anything silently in our own mind. It's a beautiful experience. And what *Devi of Speech* really means suddenly emerges, like a very clear-sounding thought. It is also at that moment where we don't feel we want to use our human voice, because our feelings are so refined, so strong, so high, that the tongue remains silent.

If there is no sound produced, you can hear what we will call "the Divine word," or the Divine sound. This leads us to mantra. And mantra is really the crown of the Devi of Speech. When chanting the Divine word, breath, vibration and rhythm are created intentionally by the use of the voice, and we begin to understand that mantra is above *all* the chatter of daily living.

Can we say that language, the Devi of Speech, is a pathway to freedom? Imagine if you don't have a voice, and you cannot express what you want to express.

How much would you be deprived of? You cannot have
a dialogue with somebody. And all that is connected
with the human voice, with words — our great plays and
epics and what-have-you — all this would be impossible.
Perhaps many things, many skills that we developed,
came about only because of the human voice: how to
make a tool, how to create something, how to build
something — it all requires communication.

  – Perhaps in the way in which we use words, there is a
certain destiny. Not the destiny of the word, but *my* or
your destiny. *Our* destiny. The use of language is a very
important thing, your awareness of that. It is a grave
mistake if we use language to reduce things to just a
collection of facts. Then language becomes some sort of
a reductionism that takes away the true value of what is
talked about. It has its purpose at some time, but that
reductionism must not enter into our daily interaction
with each other. Because it means devaluation. You may
not be aware right away that you devalue yourself as
well as others. And by that I mean how you *manipulate*
yourself, through the use of words or language. How do
you manipulate other people? When we manipulate, we

must realize there is no truth. Manipulation is pretension, a strong, powerful desire to control. But it is not truth.

The Devi of Speech as a pathway to liberation can lead you to a higher truth. It can take you from the very day of your birth to what may be your final state of liberation. How would we arrive there? That higher truth is revealed in words that are sometimes called "mantra." And when we call it "prayer," it means the communication with a force greater than our little ego. And it makes really no difference if the prayer is directed to your own soul forces, your Higher Self or the God within. However you phrase that is up to you, because it has to be your way of expression.

Words and language can be divided into the physical, the way we use language every day, and the metaphysical, which has many dimensions. We can't even say how many dimensions, for the moment, as we would have to really delve into this and explore the possibilities. Mantra is a slight indication. Prayer is. Because prayer is a conversation between you and the Divine. You petition for something. And meditation, then, means to wait in silence and emptiness of mind for the answer from the Divine forces. Perhaps we can say the Divine within, but there are also *other* forces of knowledge, other sources, that can emanate, that can reach us, if we become receptive to that.

Now if we then ask, What is the relationship of language, or the Devi of Speech to the universe? Now when we say, "Devi of Speech," perhaps we could use our more familiar term, *God*. What is God's universe?

Well, God's universe is everybody's universe, and nobody's. It depends again on how much we understand. It can be the biologist's universe, the geophysicist's universe, the astrophysicist's universe, and of course the mathematician's universe. If we keep this list going it would be a very expansive universe. And it will not tell us, however scientific our approach is, the origin of the universe. What is that Cosmic Energy? What is the Cosmic Intelligence that has all shapes and all forms and countless names, and has none?

Maybe for now, we can conclude and say, "Our universe is one of language and words."

the cakras & exercises

O Divine Mother,
May all my speech and idle talk be mantra,
All actions of my hands be mudra,
All eating and drinking be the offering
of oblations unto Thee,
All lying down prostrations before Thee.
May all pleasures be as dedicating
my entire self unto Thee.
May everything I do be taken as Thy worship.

the first cakra: muladhara

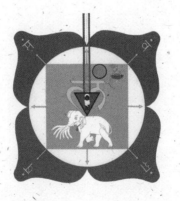

mantra for the muladhara cakra

In the Muladhara of yours I worship Him who has nine natures, dancing the great Tandava, having nine sentiments, together with (His Sakti) Samaya, the quintessence of Lasya. It is from these two, each having its own presiding form, looking in compassion on the disposition of the origination (of the world) that this world has come into existence, having you as father and mother.

commentary

In the play of the Goddess (the Devi), whose substance is consciousness, the dual principle of Siva/Sakti is presented as a male and female form, pointing to the polarity of the mind. Masculine and feminine principles are not narrowly limited, but are inseparable elements of Energy giving birth to whirling worlds, from the tiny atom to millions of galaxies. Nothing fixed, nothing rigid. Richness in mystical variations expresses life itself.

The powers of mind and matter, creation and destruction, birth and death, are an interplay of forces embodied in the dance of Tandava-Lasya. In birth, death is hidden, as heat is hidden in fire. Illusion and desire dance together. Life is a cosmic wave; dazzling creation. All forms come into existence upon the manifestation of consciousness.

the devi of muladhara

The Devi, the Goddess of Speech present in each cakra, has to be recognized as an integral part in the process of personal development.

The great significance of speech, personalized and deified, can perhaps only be understood if it is borne in mind that the ancient poets (risis) of the mantras and the Vedas (sacred texts) handed down their wisdom by word of mouth. The spoken word, trusted to memory, can float away into the distance of time because of its intangible nature. This points to the incredible power of memory of these ancient risis and their devotees that they were able to preserve perfectly the ancient scriptures.

Each letter of the Sanskrit alphabet is on a petal of the sacred cakra lotuses. This is to signify that every word or sound has power. This power is not only connected to the emotions and mental activities, but also to a Spirit of the highest order. It can, therefore, lift us to heights we ordinarily do not even anticipate. Speech has two aspects – the audible and the inaudible. Inaudible speech differs from mere talking in one's head; it is an ethereal intuitive perception. It could also be called the Language of the Heart.

The power in a word or sound is Sakti, therefore, She is called the Divine Mother in the Muladhara Cakra. She is the Goddess of Speech. On the petals of the First Cakra appear the first four letters. Because the path of Kundalini is a path of evolution, it becomes evident that with each cakra there is an increased perception of Power manifest producing all forthcoming letters.

The mere naming of things has been humankind's privilege, of which we make wide use until awareness of the true power of language is realized. Speech has to be refined. We must become aware of our speech. Sensitivity is only gained by refinement and cultivation. As a plant is cultivated, so humans must cultivate themselves to become more sensitive in a positive way. In many scriptural texts, commands or utterances can be found that seem to have the recognition of the power of the word. Its refinement and careful cultivation are reflected not only in the sacred texts, but also in the poetry of many nations. Poets, like prophets, are often ahead of their time. Some poetry has an almost prophetic nature.

Mantras are words of power and include sacred texts like the Vedas and Upanisads, formulations in praise of aspects of the Divine. On a basic level, the mantra is used as an incantation similar to those of some Christian churches. At a higher level, when it has become Mantra Yoga, the mantra is practised for single-pointedness of mind. On a still higher level, it activates and amplifies latent forces that are within every human being and that then can be termed Cosmic Forces. To speak these words or sounds of power is to acquire the power in them and to come in contact with the source of sound and thought, the "root" of the mantra.

In this cakra, Sakti Dakini holds the empty skull, representing the void, which is too awesome for the average being to conceive. The mind resists a vacuum and does its best to fill it with its own creations. So it is a constant battle to keep the mind still, in its natural state of calm (pure mind). Finally, when the mental processes have exhausted themselves through the chanting of a mantra, the mind becomes open to very subtle intuitive perceptions. At a certain point, it would not be an exaggeration to say that some of these perceptions are emanations from a source that is outside the human mind. Where and what this source is cannot be determined to the satisfaction of those who seek proof for everything.

powers of the muladhara cakra

In this cakra, we are dealing with the powerful effect of verbal and mental speech and its results on the individual mind. Self-suggestion and self-programming must be recognized to counteract their negative influence. The First Cakra is pure Energy. It is the beginning of speech, which means formulating what the childlike mind understands.

Learning is a process that goes step by step. The most intelligent level of learning is achieved when the awareness is greatest, when pride is under control, and when we can learn from our mistakes of the past, as well as from the mistakes of others, without having to repeat them. Sometimes we catch ourselves when we are just about to make a mistake, and often the awareness is there, but pride refuses to admit that the decision or action is faulty.

It is stated in the sacred texts that knowledge is eternal. This needs to be understood at a deeper level. In all ages there have lived some men and women of high intelligence and great awareness. They were able to tap the source of knowledge in themselves and by way of intuition understand the meaning of that knowledge, which they put into the language of their own time for the benefit of others. Eternal Knowledge is therefore omnipotent.

One of the promised powers of the First Cakra is Eternal Knowledge. This all-powerful knowledge requires an unusually high degree of intuitive perception.

People all over the world have the feeling that there is a Power greater than themselves. The Power is often personified but, when understood properly, the personification only applies to the vessel or the instrument through which that Power and all-powerful knowledge emanate.

Freedom from all sin is achieved at the first stage by recognizing mistakes, by controlling impulses, by learning through reflection, and by making the simultaneous connection between learning and knowledge. Sin, from a yogic point of view, is the intentional repetition of mistakes that are well-known. Mistakes that come through the process of learning are not sin. Human beings can only learn by trial and error. So again it falls to the aspirant to develop a high level of awareness and discrimination. It is within our own power to become free of sin.

Greed and ambition can deprive the mind of its wonderful potential for creativity and quality in all

aspects of living. Quality in living is the first step to
bliss. The joy of life is our inherited right. To be always
living in the spirit of gladness comes when we are free
of selfishness and all that it entails. This process of self-
mastery is indeed an experience of bliss that comes once
the early stages of learning are past.

sakti dakini

exercises for the muladhara

Speech is our most constant expression, our greatest performance and the barometer of our emotions. Between the cry for help and the cry of joy, there is a whole range of sounds expressing minute degrees of emotion. The foremost tool for self-expression is the human voice.

This cakra has only four petals, representing the first levels of speech. Remember, the energy is neutral. What do you do with it?

1 To prepare yourself for the exercises, sit comfortably and focus on the space between your eyebrows. Repeat the Divine Mother prayer aloud 25 times:

O Divine Mother,
May all my speech and idle talk be mantra,
All actions of my hands be mudra,
All eating and drinking be
offerings of oblations unto Thee,
All lying down prostrations before Thee.
May all pleasures be as dedicating
my entire self unto Thee,
May everything I do be taken as Thy worship.

Write about this experience, and your thoughts
after repeating the mantra.

2   Close your eyes. Visualize Divine Mother/the
    Devi/Sakti. What is the picture you have of
    Her in your mind?

3   Ask yourself: What is behind the urge to speak?
    Survival? Fear of silence or loneliness? Pride of
    wanting to show off what you know? Try
    keeping a ring or small coin in your mouth to
    give just enough time to ask yourself why you

need to say something and what it is you want to say, since the coin has to be tucked under the tongue or in the cheek before you can say anything.

4 Practise silence. Take a day when you do not speak, or keep silent a few hours a day for a week. Choose a time when the temptation to talk is greatest. The hours, the length of time, should be determined beforehand. Observe and record the effects.

the second cakra: svadisthana

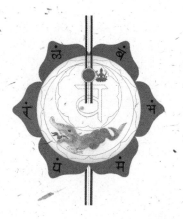

mantra for the svadisthana cakra

In the Svadisthana of yours I praise Him as Samvarta forever happy in the form of fire, O mother and also Samaya, the great one. When His glance filled with great anger consumes the worlds, it is Her glance dripping with compassion that makes this cool (soothing) service.

commentary

The Divine appears terrible only when the dark cloud of ignorance screens the seeker from consciousness. Like a child, the ignorant seeker is attracted to the toys (gadgets, money, success) of the world. In its consuming anger, Siva's powerful glance indicates that ignorance is to be burned in the fire of wisdom. It is Divine Mother's compassion that allows the truant to return and try again. This is Her most soothing service. The old ego, in spite of its struggles, has to die. The dark cloud of self-will has to be dispersed so that the Light will no longer be obscured.

the devi of svadisthana

The Devi of Speech symbolizes the first level of self-expression, and here in the Second Cakra increased refinement is already coupled with greater awareness. Awareness, when seen as a characteristic of consciousness rising or expanding to other levels of understanding, makes the idea of hierarchy of these levels more easily comprehensible. In "higher expression," language moves to a level where even meanings of words are expanded and words are used to express meanings that cannot be defined. The language of the Gods as contrasted to "ordinary language" has to be penetrated by happy listening – intuitive listening.

The same degree of intuitive perception has to be developed in listening as in speaking. This means listening within. When one listens, all mental talk has to cease – this is the state reached in true meditation. This is not to be confused with what we in the West term a state of trance, into which it is possible to slip at a certain stage of intense concentration. In meditation the mind is meant to be absolutely alert, even while it is occupied with something else. It is like a lover sitting on a bench in the park reading a book and understanding what is read, but at the same time having an inner alertness for the arrival of the beloved because the beloved is expected to come. The listening is somehow intuitively tuned in to recognizing the footsteps or the rustling of clothes, something that will announce the presence of the beloved. Immediately this is heard, the lover who waits is alert and ready to receive the beloved.

In the trance state, however, the alertness is not there and the person in trance does not perceive what the person in the true meditative state does. The lover can be so absorbed in the book that the beloved can stand in front and not be noticed. When the suggestion is given to recite or chant a mantra (it can be said that this is cultured speech and a way to cultivate the voice), it is not meant to be a trigger into a state of trance.

The meaning of every word can be stepped up to a much higher level than that which the word has in "ordinary" speech. It is up to the aspirant to cultivate perception and then to express it in a more refined way. This process should never really stop. As the intuition develops, it becomes the source of extraordinary awareness. For instance, in the beginning of musical training we learn the rhythm of a song by counting. Not so on the path of yoga. Intuitive listening is necessary to perceive the rhythm and to tune in to the teachings or to the guru. It is not a blind following, it is a slow perceiving and understanding of the why and how. When it is blind acceptance, development is so slow as to be imperceptible.

Every guru or teacher has disciples who have greater limitations than others. But it is only a question of time, patience and persistence for them to expand beyond their limitations and to become more aware and perceptive. The path is open to everyone. Only pride, the ego, greediness and self-importance prevent the aspirant from listening intuitively. Therefore the will must be applied and a clear decision made to put all else aside so that there is nothing left but full attention, listening with intuition, and surrender. When the interplay of forces between intuition and awareness has developed, listening ability will increase. The aspirant then stands on firm ground. From this direct personal experience, knowledge is gained.

Sound and its resonance are inseparable and occur in ordinary speech or song. They can give birth to powerful emotional responses. The average person misses on the very subtle level the power of sound and its resonance. The gross is not a receptacle of the subtle.

Because of our habit of naming a thing and thereby assuming that we know something about it, we find in all cultures that God has uncountable names. Each name has an inherent power because the name was created by the desire to make an immeasurable energy personal, to make it meaningful. The practising yogi or yogini tries to pull all these names together into one sound, Om.

powers of the svadisthana cakra

The ability of well-reasoned discourse or the writing of prose or verse leads to the power of imagination, which can be the basis of beautiful and inspiring words or of monster and horror stories. Writers of horror stories have often lost their minds because they did not know how to control their self-created world. The Power is neutral, and it is the responsibility of the individual how to use the imagination.

It is not possible to fully separate the powers of one cakra from another. Imagination and emotions work hand in hand, creating desires that can make almost everything possible. The image that emerges from the Second Cakra can move with lightning speed to the Third Cakra and can become a victim of the emotional impact made there. The creation of the imagination is reinforced by the emotions. Most of our fears are caused by uncultivated imagination based on ignorance. Only increased awareness can remove ignorance.

Here in the Second Cakra, the scriptural texts also say that we will be free from all enemies. It would be a mistake to personalize this and see them in the setting of the family or work situations. Rather, it is the enemies we have within ourselves, the evil inclinations driven by exerted self-will that kindle self-importance and self-absorption. Self-control is the first step, in conjunction with obedience to one's choice of the path, toward the attainment of mastery. The control of those enemies, or their destruction, will make the aspirant a sovereign among yogis and yoginis.

When one is free of all enemies and the mind dwells more steadily on the beauty of the Most High, the most ideal, that which one would like to cultivate in oneself, speech expands and another level of poetry is reached. The highest level is perhaps the poet who is also a prophet.

sakti rakini

exercises for the svadisthana

As the Lotus is sacred, the increase in the number of petals indicates an increase of expression, not only in words but, even more, in imagination. The element of water of this cakra is also symbolic of imagination. The power of imagination, the ability to arrange and rearrange images of an abstract and a concrete nature, is an extraordinary skill. How, then, is this greater ability of expression used? The aspirant should look at every action, thought or word from the point of view of *sattva* (purity), *rajas* (passion) and *tamas* (inertia) in order to further cultivate speech.

1   Close your eyes. Repeat the Divine Mother
    prayer 25 times. Visualize your Divine Mother.
    Using your imagination, describe what She looks

like. What words do you choose? Write them down. Draw a picture of your Divine Mother.

2   Investigate the connection between speech and self-image. How would you describe yourself? What words do you use? Compare them to the words you used for Divine Mother. How do you feel about your self-image? Can you nourish a new image?

3   How do impulses, strong ideas, desires, fears reflect in your speech? Look for clues in figures of speech. Ask yourself: What is tasteful to you? What is distasteful to you? Make a list and then try to explain the reasons for your responses.

4   Do a "mind-watch." Sit comfortably, with eyes closed. Watch your mind for three minutes. Note everything that comes up. Write down everything you can remember. Ask yourself: Where do thoughts come from?

the third cakra: manipura

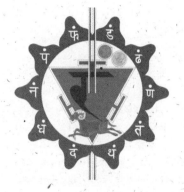

mantra for the manipura cakra

In the Manipura of yours I serve Him as a dark cloud, which is the only refuge (of the world) raining down the rain on the three worlds scorched by the sun that is Hara. (This cloud which) carries the rainbow, Indra's bow, bedecked with ornaments of various glittering jewels, and which has flashes of lightnings due to His Sakti bursting forth from the enveloping darkness (of the cloud).

commentary

The rainbow has no substance, it is intangible and cannot be grasped. The rainbow is an optical illusion that becomes perceptible to the sense of sight under certain conditions.

Sometimes the mind builds a rainbow to another dimension. Sometimes flashes of lightning (insights) glitter with jewels of intuition. Who can gaze at the sun when it is at the zenith? The light, too great, too blinding, will scorch the mind. The dark cloud offers much-needed rest, time to gather new strength.

the devi of manipura

The power of speech that has been given in the previous cakra now, in the Manipura, focuses on compulsive talking, compulsive criticism and the compulsive gratification of what are termed "needs." It must be realized that all human beings go through five stages of development: mineral-human, vegetable-human, animal-human, human-human, god-human. While it is right for us to fulfill needs in the first three groups, human-human, now in search of the path by a decision of his or her own, must look at these needs and cut them down to the essentials. Giving in to needs that should be discarded could exact a high price.

Language is born of the unconscious. The drive to express oneself comes from the unconscious. Behind many a word lies a whole range of ideas allowing numerous interpretations. For example, the words "time" and "space" spring from very different ideas when used by a housewife, an architect, a scientist, a social worker or a psychiatrist. Each profession has its particular language for specific communication with those of like mind.

Energy wasted in useless chatter is easily recognized when we are sick. We are then aware that energy is quickly depleted. There is a reluctance to conform to the social conventions that decree that one must always make talk, however small or worthless. What is the difference in the useless drain of energy in talk? If greater awareness of its preciousness does not show a purpose for the energy, then it is spilled down the drain. Observing the mind has to be carried out as an exercise to find out how it functions and to obtain greater awareness.

Changes in ourselves are frequently unnoticed. They come to the foreground, however, when attention is given to the use of words and language. In each cakra the Goddess of Speech increases. Higher levels of consciousness are approached as awareness expands. Exaggerations, superlatives, coarse language have to be left behind as one evolves; after some time, these simply drop away. The voice becomes a magnet that attracts others; the magnetism of personality comes into effect.

The scriptures speak of the Devi of Speech. The reason for giving speech a female character is that the letters of the alphabet give birth to language, to words, the sound body. They are sound symbols.

Just as complicated mathematical formulas are unintelligible to the untrained mind, so are higher aspects of the meanings of words like mantra. A magnetic/electric field is created by the chanting of mantras. The benefits are evident to those who practise Mantra Yoga. Sound has an effect on the human body in general and, in very specific ways as well, on certain limbs and organs.

powers of the manipura cakra

The power to create and destroy worlds is signified in the power of speech. How ideas are expressed, the intonation of the voice, can create an environment of blissful happiness. Self-gratification and self-glorification, with their resultant impatience, greed or pride, can destroy a harmonious relationship.

The practice of awareness by itself creates a great wealth of knowledge. In contrast to the Eternal Knowledge of the First Cakra, knowledge is now beginning to have meaning on the personal level. This is the knowledge and discrimination applied to daily events as they happen.

Appreciation of the harmonious aspects of life is personified in Sarasvati, the Goddess of Speech, of art, of music. When we can speak words of inspiration that touch an inner chord in another person, we can say that this is the worship of the Goddess Sarasvati. We thereby have created our own world of harmony in which we function.

A saintly person, by simply entering the room, can bring a sense of quiet and stillness into a tumultuous group, opening the senses of those present to higher perceptions. It is on a much higher level, and through much more training, that the worlds created by the mind can be put into words and this inner knowing of the heart can be expressed.

We have many spiritual tools that would enable us to help ourselves to a higher state of consciousness, but we allow these tools to be forgotten, the practices to become routine, and thereby never attain those other worlds of Power. The spiritual practices are too precious to be degraded to a level of routine, and in performing the exercises it is important to guard against mechanicalness if we wish to increase consciousness and attain any degree of realization.

sakti lakini (laksmi)

exercises for the manipura

In this cakra, the Manipura, we investigate the power
of the spoken word and realize that in certain respects
the power of language is not different from the power
of thought.

The Manipura Cakra, located in the region of
the navel, is the seat of the emotions. The powerful
influence of that centre on the body needs to be studied
and understood. The aspirant is probably aware of the
hypnotic effect of his or her own negative emotions. By
applying positive thinking in concrete images, this power
can be used constructively.

We can create a world of harmony, enthusiasm,
warmth when we speak words of inspiration. Through our
speech, this world can also be destroyed by negativity. How
do you use the power of speech to create and to destroy?

1 Repeat the Divine Mother prayer 25 times. Express all your longing, determination and desire to know Divine Mother. Offer all your emotions back to Her.

2 Follow a small emotional event to the root. Ask yourself: Where did it start? Why? What hooked your emotional imagination? Fear? Insecurity? Write about your experience.

3 How do I speak? Clearly? Mumbling? Do I want to be heard? Am I afraid to be heard? Is there clarity of thought? How does my voice sound when I am strong and clear? How does my voice sound when I am afraid?

4 Chant a mantra of your choice, paying attention to the breath. This links emotions with sound and is a good way to hear the emotion in your voice. This is an outlet for the restlessness caused by the emotions. The transmuting of

emotional forces into spiritual energy is
accomplished through the practice of worship.

the fourth cakra : anahata

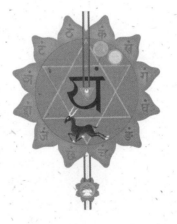

mantra for the anahata cakra

I venerate (revere, render devotional service) this pair of swans which swim in the mind of the great, feeding on the unique honey of the Lotus (heart) that is the opening of understanding. From their chatter comes the development of the eighteen kinds of knowledge, and by using them one acquires all qualities out of defects, just like taking the milk from water.

commentary

Devotion is the antidote to all self-glorification. The devotional approach includes reverence, as well as the knowing and recognizing of the Greater Power. Being devoted to Siva/Sakti, symbolized as a pair of swans in the lake of the mind, the mind becomes saturated with the milk of Divine wisdom. Through devotion the devotee opens up like the Lotus in the light of the sun. Thereby one becomes receptive to Divine knowledge, manifest in many ways. By application of this knowledge to living one is like a bee collecting honey from the flower. One emulates the swan learning to take the Divine milk from the water of illusion.

the devi of anahata

The cakras, as levels of consciousness, represent dynamic processes in people.

The Anahata Cakra controls air as well as touch. It is important to observe how speech comes about. A person who is out of breath can speak only with great difficulty. Obviously, speech without air is impossible, but the use of air, or the kind of breathing, affects speech in loudness or softness, melodiousness or abruptness. When we speak, we set up currents in the air and we are responsible for these currents.

The Sakti in this cakra holds a noose in Her hand. This warns that we can be caught not only by our emotions in speech, but by speech itself. We can love to hear ourselves talk and be caught in this infatuation. The aspirant must be committed to truth in speech and thought.

The process of clarifying the meaning of terms must be continued and, in this cakra, you will have to define such words as "consciousness" and "spiritual." This definition does not necessarily limit them, because the meaning is open to many levels of understanding.

The refinement of the senses finds its expression in speech through poetry and sometimes in prophetic poetry, because then the sound is not of the tongue but of the heart. It is like a well from which water is gently brought up from deep within. One becomes aware of the source only in those rare moments of surrender, stillness and intuition at its deepest level.

Here one may easily reach the Spirit, coming through the poetry, of a travel companion on that royal highway of spiritual life. Here the aspirant is only one step away from the communication of Selves (souls), which is beyond all words.

At this point, when the senses are refined, coarse speech is a painful experience, almost unbearable. The Devi of Speech (Sakti) is word power. Mantra is its highest expression. The sound of the voice and the vibration of it pervade the area in which the mantra is spoken. After some time, the mantra purifies the mind and the immediate orbit, which enlarges as the time of practice continues. Finally, the power of the mantra becomes a self-generating energy.

At this point it is said that the Devi, the Divine Mother, is manifest. Waves of joy and peace flood over the aspirant and a great surge of energy is experienced, expressed in most delicate, gentle feelings of devotion and surrender. The Heart is the meeting ground and some of Her Divine gifts are received here. If they are treasured and kept secret, She will be most generous. But the moment the ego puts itself on the throne that belongs to Her, the "Divine love affair" is ended. To prevent this from happening, humility has to express itself naturally; devotion to Her has to be given first place, in complete surrender. This surrender is easily attained by stilling the mind to receive Her Divine "messages," your intuitive perceptions.

The Heart Lotus is your personal temple, as indeed your whole body is. Let your mind create the atmosphere; let your feelings express that mood. Be alone when you worship in your own heart. This cakra is also called the Abode of Mercy. Mercy in feelings only is of no benefit to anyone unless this mercy is also expressed in words or actions. Mercy is forgiveness, understanding coming from the heart. As we give it, so we will receive it. There is perfect balance in the law of karma.

The Wishing Tree, the Kalpataru, is located in the Anandakanda, which lies below the Heart Lotus. We can pick the fruit from the Wishing Tree, words of sweetness and truth. This miniature Lotus is regarded as being the inner courtyard to the Anahata Cakra. It is the way of approach to the Most Holy, in an attitude of gratitude, awe and wonder. It is symbolic of the process of discovering the Divine within, and the mysteries and awesome powers of the mind. The inner courtyard then represents the experience of the manifestation of psychic energy, while the Anahata Cakra houses the tabernacle of the Most Holy from which the spiritual energies manifest.

powers of the anahata cakra

The Anahata Cakra promises the hearing with the inner ear of the cosmic *Aum*. This cosmic sound is the sound that can be heard without the striking of two objects together. It can be heard only if listening has been practised and if all the internal noises of the mind can be stopped.

The text tells us that Divine Mother Sakti dispels all fears and grants boons of the three worlds: past, present, future. If the aspirant has learned from past mistakes, the increased understanding and discrimination will mean there will be fewer mistakes in the present. The characteristics of sincerity and devotion, humility and honesty, which the aspirant will now possess from the past and the present, will somewhat determine the future, a future of harmony and happiness.

The aspirant will be able to protect this newly created environment and destroy those negative aspects that may still remain from the past. The application of what has been learned in all situations increases awareness, which takes on the soft, gentle glow of a first glimpse of what illumination could be.

By living wisely, doing noble deeds, keeping the senses under control, and having an extraordinary ability and power of concentration, the devotee or aspirant is able to render himself invisible and to enter another's body. Both of these promises need further elaboration. If I eliminate all my self-will and remove all self-protective screens, I can put myself in another's shoes and, while not identifying with the other person, I can have an understanding of that person.

To render oneself invisible, it is first necessary to overcome the desire to be in the centre of a group or to be the focus of the attention of another person. The desire for closeness to another and all the emotional needs that go with it have to be overcome first. Another person's preoccupation can also create our invisibility.

The power of concentration of one's own mind allows for the renunciation of the desire to be seen or noticed. The energy field around the body can keep the mind of a passerby suspended and make one invisible at that moment. No image of oneself is leaving the orbit of one's own energy field.

Persistent study and the practice of awareness and

discrimination will aid in acquiring these powers, but the aspirant should be warned that the results may come after many years, even lifetimes.

sakti kakini

exercises for the anahata

The Fourth Cakra is the Heart Lotus. Air and touch are the particular expressions of this cakra. The air indicates lightness; it cannot be grasped and held onto. Breathing is vital to human life. A touch as light as breath is only possible when all self-gratification has been renounced.

"Touching" and "feeling" are interchanged in everyday language. Should they be?

In the Anahata, the aspirant is at the crossroads. At this point it will be necessary to review ideals to discover if some require refining and escalating from what was originally established. This can be accomplished with the help of a review of a daily diary, which can become a valuable chart of your progress and development.

1   Repeat the Divine Mother prayer 25 times.
    Visualize Divine Mother and this time, feel
    Her presence. What does it feel like? Let Her
    come into you and fill you completely. Look at
    yourself through Her eyes of compassion. What do
    you see?

2   When have you been touched by what someone
    said? When you say that something touches your
    heart, what do you mean by this? What does it
    mean to be a friend?

3   These are four Powers of Divine Mother Sakti:

    Mahesvari: preciousness, comprehending, wisdom,
        majesty, greatness
    Mahakali: strength, will, irresistible passion
    Mahalaksmi: harmony, secrecy, compelling
        attraction, seriousness
    Mahasarasvati: perfection, intimate knowledge

    Choose one power. Ask yourself: How do I
    manifest this power?

4   Make a list of things you are grateful for in
    your life.

the fifth cakra: viśuddha

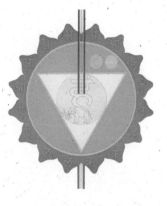

mantra for the visuddha cakra

In your Visuddha I serve Siva, the progenitor of the sky, transparent like a pure crystal, and also the Devi who is like Siva and attached to Him. It is through their beauty and graceful movements, shimmering like the rays of the moon, the world shines, its internal darkness having been dispelled, like the Cakora. (The world is feminine.)

commentary

Selfless service makes one Divine. To be a servant demands that one renounce self-will and thus become pure and transparent like the blue sky so the Divine may shine through. As the colour that gives form to the crystal cannot be separated from it, so Siva and the Devi are joined together. The graceful movements of their cosmic dance are only perceptible in those mystical moments when the ethereal inspirations are perceived like the shimmering rays of the moon, in that act of complete surrender. The Cakora bird subsists on the moonbeams. Just as it rejoices by drinking the rays of the moon, so also the *sadhaka* drinks the Brahmic bliss by meditating on Siva and Devi. The *sadhaka's* ignorance is thus dispelled.

the devi of visuddha

Speech, now refined, shows in the Fifth or Visuddha Cakra the limitations of words. Perceptions can come by thought, but these are not the highest experience. "Perception beyond words" has to be clarified. Does "beyond words" mean mental speech, or beyond mental speech? If we say "beyond mind," we must ask, "If it is beyond mind, then how can it be known?"

The Devi is the source of what is perceived beyond words, beyond mind. This is usually expressed by saying "a knowing of the heart," another dimension. Such perceptions are beyond verbalization, without colour or

form, without concepts, all-encompassing like the
sky. As an example, the rays of the sun travel in all
directions. They do not form part of the sun, but are
the sun. If consciousness is Energy (Sakti), and Energy
is indestructible, then an unusual manifestation of
consciousness can be perceived as coming through the
guru or the Devi. When the aspirant has refined the
sense of hearing to that point, this will undoubtedly be
verified by personal experience.

Speech beyond words is also saying something by a
gesture, by a touch or by an expression of the eyes.
Speaking from the heart, while audible through the use
of words, is expressing inaudibly at the same time. The
Divine Word (holy name, mantra), through the process
of practice, will become inaudible on its own account
and thus Divine speech is engendered. The power of the
spoken word is derived from a forceful desire and
therefore that power is not different from the power
of thought.

First we have the word (sound), then the vibration
of the sense that receives the sound, and third the
manifestation of what has been received. The summary

of all these ideas is expressed in the Devi of Speech. Sound and its resonance are inseparable and can result in powerful emotional responses. Beware of using words for laying a trap for others or for yourself. This can be done by asking leading questions, "putting words into the mouth" of another person. Look at your life's situation to discover where and when you have done so and which traps have already been laid. Great effort is necessary to discover these traps.

Speech that is praised is like a sweet drink or a strong spirit, bolstering the ego or the emotions. However, when the voice is the magnet that attracts others, and a chord resounds in the heart of the listener, this is a sign that the aspirant is in contact with the Devi of Speech, with Sarasvati.

From the Devi of Speech we learn that when the oil of worldly desires is burned up, She Herself, the Mother and Creatrix of all, is realized. She also tells us that unfavourable karma is burned up when Her spiritual child, the aspirant, turns the gaze fully on Her. This clears the way for the aspirant to have the strength, persistence, wisdom and circumstances necessary to achieve the goal of the full realization of the creative Energy (Kundalini). The difficulties in using everyday language to express the underlying principles make them seem almost secret. All wisdom is secret to the ignorant, and that makes it difficult to interpret such knowledge in daily language.

When we recognize that the term Devi, Divine Mother or Sakti, means Power or Intelligence at its highest, then we can speak of "Cosmic Intelligence" and see the Energy on an impersonal level.

In the Visuddha Cakra, the emphasis is on hearing. True listening means the ability to surrender, thereby speech, as well as mental talking, must be controlled in order to hear clearly. At this point it may become clearer why the Goddess of Speech appeared in each cakra and why speech is called our greatest performance. The almost insatiable need to hear ourselves talk feeds our self-importance almost to the exclusiveness even of those whom we profess to love. In the daily reflection, there should always be an entry in the diary of whether you have been able to surrender to another and how well you can stop listening to yourself. Our habitual way of hearing has to be changed in order to attain quality in listening.

The number of the petals of the Lotus is now 16, meaning that language has increased. With the development of language, humans have become more clever but unfortunately not more wise. The aspirant will find that the intellect has sharpened considerably and therefore can now cleverly talk one into or out of almost anything. Yet the aspirant is reminded that the petals belong to the Lotus, which is sacred. When all the smoke of the ego is gone and complete surrender to listening is accomplished, one can truly hear the message, be it audible or inaudible. When the clever aspects of the mind and speech are overcome, the struggle with the ensuing temptations will be less intense.

The interdependence of body and mind must also be recognized in the aspects of material (bodily), mental (abstract) and ethereal (spiritual). The aspirant will by now comprehend the use of mantra in bringing these aspects together. The practice of mantra (refined speech), the Divine Word, undergoes a process of becoming inaudible on its own account. Audible recitation improves the listening capacity and so this should be stressed rather than reciting the mantra mentally. Only when the listening capacity reaches a certain point will the mantra become self-generating.

The screens we put up to filter what we want to hear need to be removed in order to listen clearly to what others have to say and to what the inner or outer guru says. By learning to listen and by practising listening, we will know when words do not ring true, even those in our own heads.

powers of the visuddha cakra

This cakra promises that one becomes free of worldly desires. At this stage of one's life, they have served their purpose. The desires have created ambition, perfection, skills, efficiency, and helped one to see and develop strengths. The energy that is no longer locked up in the pursuit of worldly desires raises the aspirant now to a higher plane, to the Gateway of Liberation. But at the Gateway of Liberation, self-will must be surrendered to the Higher Self, no longer to the ego-mind.

All that has been learned to this point contributes to the aspirant's wealth of yoga. In the First Cakra, Eternal Knowledge has been promised and in the Third, wealth of Knowledge may be acquired. Now in the Fifth Cakra, the subjective and the objective are united in the Complete Knowledge and the aspirant comes closer to the meaning of yoga, the union.

At a later stage of development, the Complete Knowledge is all powers that can be known, or even those that are unknown except to highly developed yogis and yoginis. Complete Knowledge can only be achieved by increased concentration. The key to all powers is control of the mind. Understanding this on a deeper than intellectual level brings peace of mind that enables one to see the three worlds: the past, the present and the future. One can with greater clarity look back, see the present and anticipate the future; see what one must avoid doing, what one has to do, and perhaps what one should expand to do.

The first step in destroying danger is taken by careful thinking, the removal of all false ambition, and no longer rushing emotionally into decisions. Simply by increased awareness, greater discrimination, and more care in all actions and reactions, no longer mechanically responding to events, we understand how danger can be destroyed. This awareness creates an attitude of heart and mind that will make one merciful to all. We begin to understand that we are all a product of our environment and the victim of our own ignorance. When ignorance is removed, much danger is removed. But to become more knowing takes courage as well as a willingness to accept greater responsibility.

gauri

exercises for the visuddha

The Visuddha Cakra stands for the sense of hearing, which is, from the Western point of view, the last of the five senses. The element of the cakra, ether, means something very elusive, ethereal, and yet very powerful. To hear the Devi speak or the sound of the cosmic Aum is the crown of all experiences through the sense of hearing. This indeed may start delicately and subtly, but can become very powerful, lifting the listener into a different ethereal world.

Speech is of no relevance if there is no listener. In the Visuddha Cakra there is an ever increasing delicacy of the interaction of the energy in the body, in the mind, and in its most exercised expression of speech. Asanas are a silent manner of speech and the cells in the body, each with its own consciousness, are the listeners.

1. Repeat the Divine Mother prayer 25 times. Pay special attention to hearing yourself saying the prayer. Sit in silence for a few minutes afterward, listening. Then, ask Divine Mother a question, something you need to know from Her wisdom. Listen to Her reply.

2. Record yourself speaking. Listen to the recording and give an assessment of yourself. What do you hear?

3. Ask yourself: When I listen, what is it that listens? What do I listen to? Possible hurts? Criticism? Compliments? Can I listen to another without interrupting? Justifying? Explaining? Putting forward my point of view?

4. Investigate speech beyond words. Can you give or receive a message of love through your eyes? What other ways do you speak without using your voice?

the sixth cakra: ajna

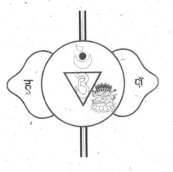

mantra for the ajna cakra

I venerate Him who is residing in the Ajna Cakra of yours. I worship (revere) the highest Sambhu in your Ajna Cakra, flanked by the highest intelligence (She), Him who has the splendour of millions of suns and moons. He who worships by propitiating with devotion will reside in the world of the Light of all lights, which is in the world, which no Earthly glance can reach and is far removed from the glance of ordinary mortals. There neither sun nor moon shines, neither fire nor the other heavenly bodies.

commentary

When mind looks at the Supreme Intelligence it stands in awe of its splendour and its Power.

The comparison of millions of suns and moons is insufficient to describe their brilliance. Even the galaxies

of stars and suns and moons can only reflect the Light
that comes from the source of all light. The Power that
has created the eye can see. The Power that created the
mind is beyond mind. Siva/Sakti is neither male nor
female (nor neuter) but existence, consciousness, bliss —
Sat-cit-ananda.

the devi of ajna

Yoga, being the path of Liberation, brings freedom
from the merry-go-round activity of the ego-mind,
strength to listen to the inner being with intuition, and
perception of the finer forces and their expression, of
which the element of this cakra, ether, is only a symbol.
Sakti, the Devi of Speech, is now understood in terms
of the language of the Gods and makes Herself known
through this inner communication, intuitive perception
and increased awareness.

   The Serpent, which has been "speechless," gently
makes its presence known and, through the Devi
of Speech, the aspirant has now acquired inner
communication, intuitive perception and an increased

awareness. Many little things seem to fall into place, or drop away. They are just gone with no struggle, no special discipline. Yet there is a strong feeling that is not entirely comfortable, a sort of fearful respect. Let that be so. Call it a holy fear. Do not slip back into old ways; always remember that your own sincerity protects you. Trust the Greater Power. Allow emotions of humility, reverence and surrender to emerge. The Serpent closes the circle. Let your intuition guide you in this thought.

The goddess Sakti-Hakini of this cakra is the creator and destroyer. This means that all personality aspects have to be killed in order that the Higher Self may live. Without destroying the old person, a new one cannot be born.

Divine Mother Sakti has to keep the world going to allow rebirth for the lessons that have not yet been learned. When you have learned all lessons, you become indeed Her child and will do Her bidding. You may also be Her special servant and offer all Energy for use as She sees fit.

If you can create Divine Mother in your mind, this is creativity of the mind at its highest. But it must also be kept alive and allowed to take its own course. You create Divine Mother in everything that is most beautiful, most perfect, most forgiving — everything that you desire to become yourself. Having created Her in your mind, you allow Her to give you energy to destroy the personality aspects that are not in keeping with this Most High creation. This makes the energy from these personality aspects available, and you put it all back into your creation of Divine Mother so that it becomes bigger, more beautiful, and, strangely enough, more real.

The two Lotus petals of this cakra represent powers that work together. They are likened to two grains of rice in which the power is compressed, but mostly unused. The lesson to be learned here is in the form of an exercise. Take a grain of rice in your hand and look at it, keeping your eyes open until they almost water. Through this process you will begin to see auras, not coloured auras, but the white aura of Light. Now you hold the rice between two fingers and hold it up to the sky.

The single-pointed mind should be directed to Siva (now properly known as Sakta) and Sakti as Power. Sakti is Power and Sakta is the source of Power — the source of Light, the Light itself. But the source will never be discovered if nothing emanates. If Light emanates, then there has to be a source from which that Energy flows. These two have to be seen together. So with the grain of rice. Without the Energy, it will not sprout. You might be able to see the Energy as an aura of life force; see the life force and the grain at the same time. This is no longer symbolic, but can be seen directly as the one Power, Sakta/Sakti.

Sakti Hakini also promises that all fears are now dispelled because of perfect Knowledge. Having reached the level of consciousness of the Sixth Cakra, one moves ever toward the Light. Excellence is now achieved with control of the mind.

The Ajna Cakra has two petals, and in the centre that connects these two petals is the complete, beautiful circle. Here again the balance of the two is that neither overrides the other, and so the control can be given to the Self, perfect in itself. The yogi calls it "resting in your own Atman." You can call it by a more familiar term, "functioning from my true Centre." The male and female aspects are shown as one. The golden dot represents the essence of all energy that will, when understood properly, hold together the two petals and let them function in perfect conjunction with each other. Here is the most powerful region of the mind, the mind being like the centre of the spheres, the indicator.

To achieve that perfect balance is not easy. Here, in the region of the mind, we have to investigate the mind to understand its functioning and purpose. And so the mind has to turn on itself. To hold the mind at bay, when it has been allowed to be the interpreter of all that passes through it for all of our lives, makes such investigation extremely difficult. The objective mind needs to be trained to raise its level of development. One method of this would be laying the foundation and building character. The second stage would be spiritual. And the combination of the two brings wisdom that we may term "celestial."

powers of the ajna cakra

At this point, the aspirant understands how one has created one's own life, all of one's pains, problems and difficulties, as a process of learning. That which has been gained needs to be preserved, and that which is no longer necessary must be destroyed. In order to fulfill the Divine union, even this perfect state in which one finds oneself, with the wisdom, the excellent powers, the pure intellect — even this state has to go as well, before the last and final plunge can be taken.

Proper identity is achieved by indeed knowing that one is created by Divine Light, or by the Cosmic Intelligence, the Absolute or God, whatever word is most desirable.

Nothing specific can be said of the excellent unknown powers of this cakra, that are mentioned in the scriptures, but the indication I can give is that there is the knowing of more than three dimensions or even four, a conception that can only be described in nebulous terms, because language has not expanded far enough for a more precise description.

Pure intellect means intellect free of selfish desires. The Śakti aspect of intellect creates. All the world is Mother Śakti's creation.

Here is, perhaps, the most crucial point where balance is needed. If the foundation has been carefully laid and all the practice done, the aspirant will have control over the powers and not be consumed by them. There will be the Divine union of the individual Self, or the individual intelligence, with the Supreme Cosmic Intelligence, by becoming half and half, male and female, intellect and intuition.

sakti hakini

exercises for the ajna

Here in the Sixth Cakra, mind has increased in subtlety and power, its mysteries becoming more comprehensible because of the work that has been done. It was an arduous task and it is not ended. The foundation has been laid for the next phase, like learning the alphabet and the grammar necessary to write the poetry that you feel is somewhere inside. There is a feeling of exhilaration in the knowing from experience — a feeling of independence.

1 Chant Om for 10 minutes. Sit in silence. Ask yourself: What is the mind? What is Consciousness? Is there a difference? Write down your reflections.

2   Before it is possible to still the mind and
    surrender, we can start on the physical level with
    Savasana or the "Death Pose."

    Lie down comfortably. Regulate the breath with
    even inhalations and exhalations. Observe how
    the rhythm creates a state of quietness and
    harmony. Become aware of your entire body.
    Starting at the feet and moving up to the head,
    ask each area of the body to relax. With each
    incoming breath, let your awareness expand.
    With each outflowing breath, relax more deeply.
    When the body is comfortably relaxed, feel the
    peace and harmony all over the body. Confirm
    that every cell is wide open to receive more of
    the great Cosmic Energy that sustains it at all
    times. Take a deep breath, open your eyes,
    stretch, move and sit up. Give gratitude for the
    gift of your body and mind.

3   Thoughts reproduce like seeds. What do you
    want to plant in your mind? Ask yourself: What

kind of person do I want to be? Make a list of the ideals you want to live by. How can you keep these ideals in mind in your daily life activities? Make a plan.

4 Write a poem about Divine Mother. Describe Her as everything that is most beautiful, most perfect, most forgiving — everything you desire to become yourself.

divine mother's grace

Sakti, your body is the World.
The rivers are your veins,
And the forest, your hair.
The firmament is your dress.
The mind is your breath.
You are the pairs of opposites.
You are the past and the present,
The soft and the gentle,
The terrible and the fierce.
Your sounds are silence.
You are waves of sound,
And the power of silence.
You are the human and the Divine.
You are elevated places, the labyrinth,
The one without a second.
O Mother of many aspects.

the last illusion

On the path to Liberation from illusion, the relationship of the aspirant to Divine Mother must be built on the firm foundation of good character, self-discipline and a faith that ever deepens. Eventually, when this faith is no longer blind, the aspirant knows within the heart the presence of Divine Mother, and an intimate play of forces follows, which no verbalization can truly express. The description "living in Divine Mother's grace" fits perfectly.

As long as the aspirant keeps the contact with Her, She will take care of Her Divine child with a love and a tenderness unknown before. Life takes on a new meaning.

The kind of life one decides to live is up to the individual. After obtaining Her grace, an aspirant may not want to grow more into Her Light, but may desire to resume previous activities with another dimension. Another aspirant, having once tasted Her Divine nectar, may become an inspiration to others and continue to expand in the desire for a higher state of consciousness. Another may perfectly surrender to Her and desire nothing more than to be led by Her, wherever She takes Her Divine child (servant).

If She is wanted for Herself, all illusion comes to an end, and so does pain. It sounds easy and yet it seems to be, and really is, a constant battle against the stream of life. Life is not to be rejected, but to be transformed.

The last illusion is Sakti Herself.

bibliography

Avalon, Arthur (Sir John Woodroffe). *Garland of Letters*. India: Nesma Books, 2001.

———— and Ellen Avalon. *Hymns to the Goddess and Hymn to Kali*. Madras, India: Ganesh & Co., 2001.

Brown, C. Mackenzie. *Devi Gita: Song of the Goddess*. Albany, NY: SUNY Press, 1998.

————. *God As Mother: A Feminine Theology in India*. Hartford, VT: Claude Stark, 1974.

Guenther, Herbert V. *The Tantric View of Life*. Boston: Shambhala Publications, 1976.

Hixon, Lex. *Mother of the Buddhas*. Wheaton, IL: Quest Books, 1993.

Shankaranarayanan, S. *Glory of the Divine Mother*. Veyangoda, Sri Lanka: Prabha Publishers, 2001.

Sivananda, Swami (trans.). *Ananda Lahari (The Wave of Bliss)*. Calcutta, India: The S.P. League, 1949.

Tulku, Tarthang (trans.). *Mother of Knowledge: The Enlightenment of Yeshe Tsogyal*. Berkeley, CA: Dharma Publishing, 1983.

contact us

🪷 timeless books
www.timeless.org

in Canada:
p.o. box 9 Kootenay Bay, BC   VOB IXO
contact@timeless.org   800.661.8711

in the United States:
p.o. box 3543, Spokane, WA   99220-3543
info@timeless.org   800.251.9273

about the author

swami sivananda radha (1911–1995) authored more
than 10 books on yoga and spirituality, including the
classic *Kundalini Yoga for the West*, and *Radha: Diary of a
Woman's Search*. She is the founder of Yasodhara Ashram,
and the inspiration for the award-winning yoga
magazine, *ascent*. She is known for her practical and
passionate teachings, which are an intrinsic part of the
yogic tradition in the West. For more information on
Swami Sivananda Radha and her teachings, visit
www.yasodhara.org.